BLADDER CANCER

Causes, Diagnosis, Treatment, and Survivorship Strategies

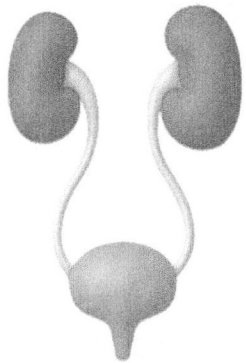

Dr. Catherine Davis

Copyright © 2024 by Dr. Catherine Davis

All rights reserved.

No part of this publication may be reproduced, distributed, or transmitted in any form or by any means, including photocopying, recording, or other electronic or mechanical methods, without the prior written permission of the publisher, except in the case of brief quotations embodied in critical reviews and certain other noncommercial uses permitted by copyright law.

Table of Contents

Table of Contents 3

Introduction 5

    Understanding the Bladder 5

    Overview of Bladder Cancer 6

Chapter 1: Causes and Risk Factors 9

    Genetic Factors 9

    Environmental Factors 10

    Lifestyle Factors 12

Chapter 2: Signs and Symptoms 15

    Early Warning Signs 15

    Advanced Symptoms 17

    Diagnostic Tests 19

Chapter 3: Types and Stages of Bladder Cancer 23

    Non-Invasive Bladder Cancer 23

    Invasive Bladder Cancer 25

    Staging Systems 27

Chapter 4: Treatment Options 31

    Surgery 31

    Chemotherapy 33

    Immunotherapy 34

Radiation Therapy 36
Targeted Therapy 37
Chapter 5: Managing Side Effects 41
Coping with Treatment Side Effects............................. 41
Supportive Care 44
Chapter 6: Living with Bladder Cancer 47
Lifestyle Modifications 47
Emotional Well-being... 50
Support Resources 52
Chapter 7: Survivorship and Follow-Up Care 55
Long-Term Monitoring... 55
Preventive Measures... 58
Recurrence Management 60
Chapter 8: Advances in Bladder Cancer Research............ 63
Emerging Therapies.. 63
Clinical Trials 66
Chapter 9: Personal Stories of Hope and Resilience......... 71
Patient Perspectives.. 71
Caregiver Experiences.. 74
Conclusion 79

Introduction

Understanding the Bladder

The bladder, a hollow organ found in the pelvis, plays a critical role in the urinary system. Its principal purpose is to hold urine produced by the kidneys before elimination. Structurally, the bladder is formed of multiple layers of tissue, including the inner lining called the urothelium, muscle layers, and outside connective tissue.

During urination, the bladder muscles contract, releasing urine through the urethra. This mechanism is regulated by a complicated interplay of nerves and muscles, guaranteeing efficient bladder function. Any interruption to this sophisticated system can lead to many bladder-related disorders, including infections, urine incontinence, and, most notably, bladder cancer.

Overview of Bladder Cancer

Bladder cancer is a tumor that develops in the cells of the bladder lining. It is one of the most frequent malignancies affecting the urinary system, with thousands of new cases detected each year worldwide. While bladder cancer can develop at any age, it is more prevalent in older persons, particularly those over the age of 55.

The exact cause of bladder cancer is generally complicated, involving a combination of genetic predisposition, environmental exposures, and lifestyle factors. Chronic exposure to some carcinogens, such as tobacco smoke, industrial chemicals, and certain pharmaceuticals, has been associated with an increased chance of developing bladder cancer.

Bladder cancer generally manifests with symptoms such as blood in the urine (hematuria), frequent urination, pain during urination, and pelvic discomfort. However, early-stage bladder cancer may be asymptomatic and identified incidentally during normal medical tests or screenings.

The diagnosis of bladder cancer usually involves a combination of medical history review, physical examination, imaging techniques (such as ultrasound, CT scan, or MRI), and urinary testing (including urine cytology and urine culture). Definitive diagnosis sometimes involves a technique called cystoscopy, in which a thin, flexible tube with a camera is introduced into the bladder to examine any abnormalities and collect tissue samples for biopsy.

Once identified, the treatment approach for bladder cancer depends on numerous aspects, including the stage and grade of the cancer, as well as the patient's overall health and preferences. Treatment options may include surgery, chemotherapy, immunotherapy, radiation therapy, or a combination of these methods.

Despite substantial breakthroughs in treatment choices, bladder cancer can be tough to manage, particularly in situations of advanced or recurring disease. Therefore, ongoing research efforts focus on establishing novel therapy options, improving early detection tools, and better overall patient outcomes.

In the following parts, we will look deeper into the causes, risk factors, signs and symptoms, diagnostic tools, treatment options, and survivorship measures connected to bladder cancer, seeking to provide thorough insights into this complicated disease.

Chapter 1: Causes and Risk Factors

Genetic Factors

Genetic factors have a key influence in predisposing individuals to bladder cancer. Several genetic abnormalities and variants have been identified that can enhance an individual's propensity to develop bladder cancer. These genetic changes may disrupt multiple biological pathways involved in cell development, proliferation, and DNA repair systems.

For example, mutations in genes encoding for proteins involved in DNA repair mechanisms, such as the tumor suppressor genes TP53 and RB1, have been implicated in bladder cancer growth. Additionally, changes in genes associated with cell cycle regulation, apoptosis, and immune response pathways may contribute to the initiation and progression of bladder cancer.

Family history also plays a key role in determining bladder cancer risk. Individuals with a first-degree family (parent, sibling, or child) who have had bladder cancer are at an elevated risk of acquiring the disease themselves. This shows a potential hereditary component to bladder cancer susceptibility, however particular genetic mechanisms causing familial bladder cancer instances are still being explored.

Environmental Factors

Environmental exposures to carcinogenic chemicals are substantial risk factor for bladder cancer development. Occupational exposure to certain chemicals and poisons is particularly noteworthy in this regard. Workers in industries such as rubber manufacture, textile dyeing, chemical production, and printing have an enhanced risk of bladder cancer due to exposure to chemicals including aromatic amines, benzene, and arsenic.

Cigarette smoking is another well-established environmental risk factor for bladder cancer. Tobacco smoke contains various carcinogens, including aromatic amines and polycyclic aromatic hydrocarbons, which can be absorbed into the bloodstream and eliminated in urine. These carcinogens come into close touch with the bladder lining, increasing the likelihood of DNA damage and malignant transformation of bladder cells.

Other environmental factors related to bladder cancer risk include exposure to certain drugs, such as cyclophosphamide and phenacetin, as well as recurrent urinary tract infections and bladder inflammation. Additionally, ingestion of contaminated water and exposure to arsenic in drinking water have been associated with an increased risk of bladder cancer in particular geographic regions.

Lifestyle Factors

Several lifestyle variables have been implicated in the development of bladder cancer. Poor dietary habits, typified by poor intake of fruits and vegetables and heavy consumption of processed foods, may contribute to an increased risk of bladder cancer. A diet rich in antioxidants and phytochemicals has been found to have preventive benefits against cancer development, including bladder cancer.

Chronic dehydration and poor fluid intake may potentially play a role in bladder cancer risk. Insufficient hydration can lead to concentrated urine, which may increase the concentration and length of exposure of bladder cells to carcinogens present in the urine.

Furthermore, obesity and physical inactivity have been related to an enhanced risk of bladder cancer. Adipose tissue releases inflammatory cytokines and hormones that can encourage tumor growth and progression. Additionally, persons who are overweight or obese may have abnormalities in insulin signaling pathways, which might lead to cancer development.

Bladder cancer is a complex illness driven by a mix of hereditary, environmental, and lifestyle factors. Understanding these risk factors is vital for implementing preventative measures and creating tailored interventions to lessen the burden of bladder cancer on individuals and society as a whole.

14 | BLADDER CANCER

Chapter 2: Signs and Symptoms

Early Warning Signs

Recognizing the early warning signals of bladder cancer is critical for rapid diagnosis and treatment. While symptoms may vary from person to person, some frequent early markers include:

1. Hematuria (Blood in Urine): One of the most prevalent early indications of bladder cancer is the presence of blood in the urine (hematuria). This may appear as pink, crimson, or cola-colored urine and can occur occasionally or frequently.

2. Changes in urine patterns: Individuals with bladder cancer may suffer changes in their urine patterns, such as increased frequency of urination, urgency (sudden and intense urge to urinate), and dysuria (painful urination).

3. Pelvic Pain or Discomfort: Some persons may have pelvic pain or discomfort, which can range from mild to severe and may be chronic or intermittent.

4. Urinary Tract Infections (UTIs): Recurrent urinary tract infections, especially in the absence of other risk factors, may be an early indicator of bladder cancer. UTIs that do not respond to routine therapies or occur frequently should urge further assessment.

5. Unexplained Weight Loss: In some circumstances, unexplained weight loss may occur as a result of cancer-related metabolic changes or reduced appetite owing to discomfort or suffering.

Advanced Symptoms

As bladder cancer grows, symptoms may become more prominent and may include:

1. Severe Hematuria: Advanced bladder cancer may cause substantial bleeding into the urine, resulting in visible blood clots or anemia (low red blood cell count).

2. Painful Urination: As the tumor grows and obstructs the urinary tract, patients may suffer increased discomfort or burning sensation during urination.

3. Pelvic or Back Pain: Advanced bladder cancer can produce pelvic or back pain that may intensify over time and may be accompanied by other symptoms such as bone pain (if cancer has spread to the bones).

4. Urinary Obstruction: In some circumstances, bladder cancer may restrict the flow of urine, resulting in urinary retention (inability to empty the bladder fully), which can cause discomfort and raise the risk of urinary tract infections.

5. Swelling in the Lower Legs: Swelling (edema) in the lower legs may occur if bladder cancer obstructs the flow of urine, resulting in fluid retention and impaired kidney function.

Diagnostic Tests

Several diagnostic tests may be done to evaluate persons with suspected bladder cancer. These may include:

1. Urinalysis: A simple urine test can reveal the presence of blood, abnormal cells, or other compounds that may suggest bladder cancer.

2. Imaging Studies: Imaging tests such as ultrasonography, computed tomography (CT) scan, magnetic resonance imaging (MRI), or intravenous pyelogram (IVP) may be used to examine the bladder and surrounding structures and detect any abnormalities.

3. Cystoscopy: A cystoscopy is a technique in which a thin, flexible tube containing a camera (cystoscope) is introduced into the bladder through the urethra. This allows the clinician to directly visualize the inside of the bladder and do a biopsy (tissue sample) if any abnormalities are identified.

4. Biopsy: During cystoscopy, a tissue sample (biopsy) may be obtained from questionable locations within the bladder for further examination under a microscope. This helps confirm the diagnosis of bladder cancer and define its kind and stage.

5. Urine Cytology: Urine cytology includes examining urine samples under a microscope to check for abnormal cells shed from the lining of the bladder. While not as sensitive as other tests, urine cytology can aid in the detection of bladder cancer, especially in cases with high-grade tumors.

Recognizing the signs and symptoms of bladder cancer, especially in its early stages, is critical for timely diagnosis and treatment. Diagnostic tests play a significant role in verifying the presence of bladder cancer and guiding optimal therapy choices. Early detection and care can dramatically improve results for persons affected by this condition.

Chapter 3: Types and Stages of Bladder Cancer

Non-Invasive Bladder Cancer

Non-invasive bladder cancer refers to tumors that are restricted to the inner lining of the bladder (urothelium) and have not infiltrated the muscular layer or adjacent tissues. This form of bladder cancer is often classed as either non-muscle invasive bladder cancer (NMIBC) or carcinoma in situ (CIS).

1. **Non-Muscle Invasive Bladder Cancer (NMIBC):** NMIBC accounts for the majority of bladder cancer cases and includes tumors that are restricted to the urothelium (innermost layer of the bladder). These tumors may be classed as low-grade or high-grade based on their aggressiveness and likelihood of recurrence and progression.

- **Low-grade Ta/T1 tumors:** These tumors are usually slow-growing and have a lower risk of recurrence and progression. Treatment may involve transurethral resection of the bladder tumor (TURBT), followed by intravesical therapy (instillation of chemotherapy or immunotherapy drugs into the bladder) to lower the chance of recurrence.

- **High-grade Ta/T1 tumors:** High-grade tumors are more aggressive and have a higher chance of recurrence and progression to invasive disease. Treatment often involves TURBT followed by intravesical treatment or, in rare cases, early cystectomy (surgical removal of the bladder) to avoid disease progression.

2. Carcinoma in Situ (CIS): CIS is a high-grade form of non-invasive bladder cancer defined by the presence of aberrant cells restricted to the urothelium. While CIS does not penetrate the bladder muscle, it has a significant chance of advancing to invasive illness if left untreated. Treatment may comprise intravesical treatment or early cystectomy, depending on the extent and aggressiveness of the disease.

Invasive Bladder Cancer

Invasive bladder cancer refers to cancers that have breached the muscle layer of the bladder wall and may expand into surrounding tissues or organs. This kind of bladder cancer is more aggressive and carries a higher chance of metastasis (spread to other regions of the body). Invasive bladder cancer is often divided into numerous subgroups based on the extent of invasion and histological characteristics.

1. Muscle-Invasive Bladder Cancer (MIBC): MIBC accounts for a smaller percentage of bladder cancer patients but is associated with a poorer prognosis compared to non-invasive disease. These tumors have penetrated the muscle layer of the bladder wall and may expand into neighboring tissues such as the prostate, uterus, or pelvic wall. Treatment for MIBC frequently entails radical cystectomy (surgical removal of the bladder) with or without preoperative chemotherapy or radiation therapy.

2. Metastatic Bladder Cancer: Metastatic bladder cancer occurs when cancer cells move from the bladder to distant organs or lymph nodes. Common locations of metastasis include the lymph nodes, liver, lungs, and bones. Metastatic bladder cancer is associated with a drastically reduced life expectancy and requires systemic therapy, such as chemotherapy, immunotherapy, or targeted therapy, to manage the disease and improve quality of life.

Staging Systems

Staging systems are used to diagnose bladder cancer depending on the extent of disease dissemination and guide treatment options. The two most often used staging methods for bladder cancer are the TNM staging system and the American Joint Committee on Cancer (AJCC) staging system.

1. TNM Staging System: The TNM staging system classifies bladder cancer based on three major factors: Tumor size and invasion (T), lymph node involvement (N), and distant metastases (M). Tumors are graded from Ta (non-invasive) to T4 (invasive), with additional subcategories indicating the level of tumor invasion and spread.

2. AJCC Staging System: The AJCC staging system integrates information from the TNM staging system to assign an overall stage grouping to bladder cancer. Stages vary from 0 (non-invasive) to IV (metastatic), with further subdivisions based on tumor size, lymph node involvement, and distant metastasis.

Accurate staging of bladder cancer is critical for assessing prognosis and directing therapy decisions. Multidisciplinary evaluation and staging may entail a combination of imaging scans, cystoscopy, biopsy, and other diagnostic testing to assess the amount of disease dissemination and adjust treatment regimens to individual patient needs. Early detection and early management of bladder cancer are crucial for improving outcomes and maximizing survival rates for affected patients.

30 | BLADDER CANCER

Chapter 4: Treatment Options

Surgery

Surgery is the main treatment option for bladder cancer, particularly for localized disease or situations where the tumor has entered the muscle layer of the bladder wall. Several surgical methods may be performed based on the stage and scope of the cancer:

1. Transurethral Resection of Bladder Tumor (TURBT): TURBT is a minimally invasive technique performed utilizing a cystoscope introduced through the urethra. It is used to remove non-invasive or superficial bladder cancers and obtain tissue samples for biopsy.

2. Partial Cystectomy: In certain cases where the tumor is restricted to a small section of the bladder wall, a part of the bladder may be surgically removed while preserving bladder function.

3. Radical Cystectomy: Radical cystectomy entails the surgical removal of the entire bladder, neighboring lymph nodes, and surrounding organs (such as the prostate or uterus) in cases of aggressive bladder cancer. Urinary diversion treatments, such as ileal conduit or neobladder reconstruction, are performed to reroute urine flow and maintain urinary continence.

4. Pelvic Lymph Node Dissection: Lymph node dissection may be performed concurrently with cystectomy to remove neighboring lymph nodes and assess for spread of malignancy.

Chemotherapy

Chemotherapy is a systemic treatment strategy that involves the use of chemicals to eliminate cancer cells or stop their growth. It may be delivered before or after surgery, depending on the stage and severity of the malignancy. Chemotherapy may be used in the following ways:

1. Neoadjuvant Chemotherapy: Administered before surgery, neoadjuvant chemotherapy seeks to reduce the tumor, making it more operable and minimizing the likelihood of disease recurrence.

2. Adjuvant Chemotherapy: Given after surgery, adjuvant chemotherapy helps to eliminate any leftover cancer cells and lowers the risk of cancer recurrence.

3. Chemotherapy for Advanced Disease: In cases of metastatic or unresectable bladder cancer, chemotherapy may be administered as the primary treatment to manage the disease, reduce symptoms, and enhance quality of life.

Immunotherapy

Immunotherapy utilizes the body's immune system to recognize and fight cancer cells. The main kind of immunotherapy utilized for bladder cancer is immune checkpoint inhibitors, which block proteins that suppress the immune response. Key drugs utilized in immunotherapy for bladder cancer include:

1. PD-1/PD-L1 Inhibitors: Drugs such as pembrolizumab, nivolumab, and atezolizumab target the PD-1/PD-L1 pathway to boost immune system activation against bladder cancer cells.

2. Bacillus Calmette-Guérin (BCG) Therapy: BCG is a form of immunotherapy used for non-muscle invasive bladder cancer. It is given directly into the bladder to trigger an immune response and prevent cancer recurrence.

Immunotherapy has transformed the treatment landscape for bladder cancer, particularly for advanced illnesses where standard treatments may be unsuccessful.

Radiation Therapy

Radiation therapy uses high-energy beams to kill cancer cells or shrink tumors. It may be used alone or in combination with surgery or chemotherapy for bladder cancer treatment. Radiation therapy for bladder cancer may involve:

1. External Beam Radiation Therapy (EBRT): EBRT distributes radiation from outside the body using a machine, targeting the tumor and surrounding tissues.

2. Brachytherapy: Brachytherapy involves the insertion of radioactive sources directly into or around the tumor, providing high doses of radiation to the cancer location while minimizing exposure to surrounding healthy tissues.

Radiation therapy may be used as a primary treatment for bladder cancer in cases where surgery is not viable or as a palliative treatment to relieve symptoms and enhance the quality of life in advanced illness.

Targeted Therapy

Targeted therapy focuses on specific molecular targets implicated in cancer growth and progression. While not yet as frequently utilized as other therapy techniques for bladder cancer, targeted therapies show potential in specific cases, particularly for advanced or metastatic disease. Targeted therapy options for bladder cancer may include:

1. **FGFR Inhibitors:** Drugs targeting fibroblast growth factor receptor (FGFR) mutations or changes, such as erdafitinib, are being studied for the treatment of advanced bladder cancer.

2. **EGFR Inhibitors:** Epidermal growth factor receptor (EGFR) inhibitors, such as cetuximab, may be administered in combination with chemotherapy for certain individuals with metastatic bladder cancer.

3. **PI3K/AKT/mTOR Inhibitors:** Inhibitors of the PI3K/AKT/mTOR pathway are being examined in clinical trials for their potential involvement in treating bladder cancer, particularly in patients resistant to conventional therapy.

Bladder cancer treatment choices continue to change, with advancements in surgery, chemotherapy, immunotherapy, radiation therapy, and targeted therapy bringing new hope for patients. Multidisciplinary teamwork and tailored treatment techniques are critical to enhance results and improve the quality of life for persons affected with bladder cancer.

Chapter 5: Managing Side Effects

Coping with Treatment Side Effects

Managing side effects is a critical element of cancer treatment, especially bladder cancer therapy. While therapy side effects can vary based on the individual modality employed, there are several common ways of coping with them:

1. Open contact: Maintain open and honest contact with your healthcare provider about any side effects you experience. They can provide direction, and support, and even change your treatment plan to minimize discomfort.

2. Symptom Management: Work with your healthcare provider to manage particular side effects such as nausea, exhaustion, discomfort, and urine difficulties. Medications, lifestyle adjustments, and supportive therapies (e.g., acupuncture, massage) may be prescribed to alleviate symptoms.

3. Nutrition and Hydration: Maintain a balanced diet rich in nutrients to support your overall health and well-being during treatment. Stay hydrated by drinking plenty of fluids, but avoid alcohol and caffeine, which can irritate the bladder.

4. Physical Activity: Engage in frequent physical activity as tolerated to help overcome fatigue, boost mood, and maintain strength and endurance. Consult with your healthcare team before starting any fitness routine, and adapt activities based on your energy levels and treatment side effects.

5. Emotional help: Seek emotional help from friends, family, support groups, or mental health specialists to cope with the emotional problems of bladder cancer diagnosis and treatment. Sharing your feelings and experiences with those who understand can bring comfort and insight.

6. Mind-Body Techniques: Practice relaxation techniques such as deep breathing, meditation, yoga, or guided imagery to reduce stress, and anxiety, and increase overall well-being. These approaches can help you cope with treatment-related challenges and build your resilience.

7. Self-Care: Prioritize self-care activities that bring you comfort and joy, whether it's spending time with loved ones, pursuing hobbies, or engaging in creative outlets. Taking care of your emotional and psychological needs is equally as vital as controlling physical side effects.

Supportive Care

Supportive care plays a key role in minimizing side effects and enhancing the quality of life for persons receiving bladder cancer therapy. Here are some supportive care measures widely used:

1. Pain Management: If you have pain due to bladder cancer or its treatment, your healthcare team can prescribe drugs or other measures to assist in alleviating discomfort and improve your quality of life.

2. Dietary Support: A certified dietitian can give tailored dietary counsel to help you maintain adequate food intake, manage treatment-related side effects (such as nausea and taste changes), and support general health and well-being.

3. Physical Therapy: Physical therapists can offer exercises, stretches, and strategies to improve mobility, strength, and function during and after bladder cancer treatment. They can also address particular disorders such as urinary incontinence or pelvic floor dysfunction.

4. Psychosocial Support: Psychosocial support services, including counseling, support groups, and resources for coping with stress, anxiety, and depression, can help you manage the emotional obstacles of bladder cancer diagnosis and treatment.

5. Palliative Care: Palliative care doctors focus on reducing symptoms, managing pain, and enhancing the quality of life for persons with serious illnesses such as bladder cancer. Palliative care can be delivered with curative treatment and is not restricted to end-of-life care.

6. Continued Monitoring and Follow-Up: Regular follow-up consultations with your healthcare team are critical for monitoring treatment response, managing side effects, and resolving any new or persistent issues. These appointments allow for continuing assessment and revision of your care plan as needed.

Minimizing side effects and providing supportive care are key components of bladder cancer treatment.

Chapter 6: Living with Bladder Cancer

Lifestyle Modifications

Living with bladder cancer frequently entails making lifestyle alterations to maximize health, manage symptoms, and support overall well-being. Here are some lifestyle adjustments that may benefit patients with bladder cancer:

1. Quit Smoking: If you smoke, quitting is one of the most essential acts you can do to improve your health and lower the risk of cancer recurrence. Smoking cessation can also boost the efficiency of bladder cancer treatment and lower the risk of problems.

2. Healthy Diet: Adopting a balanced diet rich in fruits, vegetables, whole grains, and lean proteins can supply necessary nutrients and support general health. Limiting processed meals, red meat, and alcohol consumption may also be advantageous.

3. Stay Hydrated: Drinking enough fluids, particularly water, can assist in maintaining hydration and support bladder health. However, persons with bladder cancer may need to avoid some beverages (such as alcohol, caffeine, and citrus juices) that might irritate the bladder and increase symptoms.

4. Exercise Regularly: Engaging in regular physical activity, such as walking, swimming, or yoga, can help increase energy levels, reduce stress, and enhance overall well-being. Talk to your healthcare staff about appropriate exercise options based on your health status and treatment plan.

5. Manage Stress: Chronic stress can significantly damage physical and emotional health, so finding effective stress management techniques is crucial. Relaxation techniques, mindfulness meditation, and engaging in enjoyable activities can help decrease stress and promote relaxation.

6. Maintain a Healthy Weight: Maintaining a healthy weight through diet and exercise can help lower the chance of cancer recurrence, enhance treatment outcomes, and support overall health and well-being.

Emotional Well-being

Emotional well-being is a critical element of living with bladder cancer and can dramatically affect quality of life. Coping with the emotional problems of a cancer diagnosis involves support, perseverance, and self-care. Here are some ways to enhance emotional well-being:

1. Seek Support: Connect with friends, family members, support groups, or mental health experts who can provide empathy, understanding, and practical support. Sharing your feelings and experiences with people who have gone through similar situations may be reassuring and empowering.

2. Practice Self-Care: Prioritize self-care activities that promote relaxation, enjoyment, and self-compassion. Engage in activities that bring you delight, whether it's spending time outdoors, pursuing hobbies, or practicing mindfulness meditation.

3. Stay educated: Educate yourself about bladder cancer, treatment options, and self-care practices to empower yourself and make educated decisions about your health care. However, be aware of information overload and seek credible sources of information.

4. Express Yourself: Expressing your thoughts, feelings, and concerns through journaling, painting, or creative activities can be therapeutic and help you process emotions linked to your cancer journey.

5. Address Mental Health Needs: If you're experiencing signs of anxiety, depression, or other mental health difficulties, don't hesitate to get expert help. Mental health specialists can give counseling, therapy, or medication management to assist your emotional well-being.

Support Resources

Accessing support resources and services can provide practical aid, knowledge, and emotional support throughout your bladder cancer journey. Here are some resources to consider:

1. Cancer Support Organizations: Organizations such as the American Cancer Society, CancerCare, and the Bladder Cancer Advocacy Network (BCAN) offer a wide range of resources, including educational materials, support groups, and financial aid programs.

2. Online Communities: Online forums, social media groups, and virtual support communities allow chances to interact with other individuals impacted by bladder cancer, share experiences, and offer mutual support.

3. Patient Navigators: Patient navigators or oncology social workers can assist you navigate the healthcare system, locating resources, and coordinating care throughout your bladder cancer treatment journey.

4. Clinical Trials: Clinical trials offer access to breakthrough therapies and research opportunities for persons with bladder cancer. Talk to your healthcare team about whether participation in a clinical study may be appropriate for you.

5. Supportive Care Services: Palliative care and supportive care services focus on treating symptoms, enhancing quality of life, and addressing psychosocial needs for patients with cancer and their families.

Living with bladder cancer requires a holistic strategy that covers physical, emotional, and practical concerns. By making lifestyle modifications, prioritizing mental well-being, and accessing support networks, persons with bladder cancer can enhance their quality of life and navigate their cancer experience with resilience and empowerment.

Chapter 7: Survivorship and Follow-Up Care

Long-Term Monitoring

Survivorship and follow-up care are crucial components of the continuum of care for persons who have finished treatment for bladder cancer. Long-term monitoring comprises regular follow-up consultations with healthcare experts to check for recurrence, manage late effects of therapy, and address ongoing health concerns. Here are some critical components of long-term surveillance for bladder cancer survivors:

1. Follow-up program: Your healthcare team will develop a follow-up program based on the stage and type of bladder cancer, treatment received, and individual risk factors. Follow-up appointments may initially be more frequent and gradually spaced out over time.

2. Physical Examinations: Regular physical examinations, including pelvic exams and probing of the abdomen, help healthcare providers monitor for any signs of recurrence or advancement of bladder cancer. Your healthcare team may also undertake standard blood tests and imaging examinations as part of the evaluation.

3. Cystoscopy: Cystoscopy is an important method for monitoring bladder cancer recurrence. Follow-up cystoscopies may be conducted at regular intervals to visualize the inside of the bladder and examine for any abnormal growths or changes in the bladder lining.

4. Imaging examinations: Depending on your unique circumstances, imaging examinations such as CT scans, MRI scans, or ultrasound may be indicated to assess the bladder, kidneys, and surrounding structures for any evidence of recurrence or metastasis.

5. Urinary Tests: Periodic urine tests, including urine cytology and urinalysis, may be undertaken to detect any abnormal cells or symptoms of bladder cancer recurrence.

6. Symptom Monitoring: Pay attention to any new or persistent symptoms such as blood in the urine, urinary changes, pelvic pain, or unexplained weight loss. Promptly report any concerned symptoms to your healthcare team for further investigation.

Preventive Measures

In addition to frequent monitoring, bladder cancer survivors can make proactive efforts to lower the chance of cancer recurrence and promote general health and well-being. Here are some preventive steps to consider:

1. Smoking Cessation: If you smoke, quitting smoking is one of the most essential steps you can take to lower the chance of bladder cancer recurrence and improve overall health. Avoid exposure to secondhand smoke and other environmental toxins wherever feasible.

2. Healthy Lifestyle: Adopting a healthy lifestyle that includes frequent exercise, a balanced diet, and keeping a healthy weight will help lower the chance of cancer recurrence and improve overall health. Aim for a diet rich in fruits, vegetables, whole grains, and lean proteins, and minimize processed foods, red meat, and alcohol consumption.

3. **Stay Hydrated:** Drinking plenty of fluids, particularly water, can assist in maintaining urinary tract health and lower the chance of bladder discomfort or infection. Aim to consume at least eight glasses of water every day, and avoid excessive use of caffeine, alcohol, and other bladder irritants.

4. **Sun Protection:** Protect your skin from sun exposure by using sunscreen, protective clothes, and seeking shade when outdoors. Individuals who have undergone bladder cancer therapy may be at increased risk of acquiring some skin malignancies, thus sun protection is very necessary.

5. Regular Medical Check-ups: Attend regular follow-up meetings with your healthcare team and participate in recommended cancer screening tests, such as colonoscopies or mammograms, as indicated depending on your age, gender, and specific risk factors.

Recurrence Management

Despite the best preventive measures, bladder cancer recurrence can occur. If cancer does reappear, it's crucial to swiftly address it with suitable therapy and care measures. Here are some considerations for managing bladder cancer recurrence:

1. Treatment Options: The treatment approach for recurrent bladder cancer depends on numerous aspects, including the location and extent of recurrence, previous treatments taken, and individual health status. Treatment options may include surgery, chemotherapy, immunotherapy, radiation therapy, or a combination of these methods.

2. Clinical Trials: Consider enrolling in clinical trials testing innovative medicines or therapeutic methods for recurrent bladder cancer. Clinical trials offer access to breakthrough medicines and research possibilities that may improve outcomes for individuals with recurrent disease.

3. Multidisciplinary Care: Seek care from a multidisciplinary team of healthcare specialists with expertise in managing bladder cancer recurrence. Your treatment plan may entail coordination between urologists, medical oncologists, radiation oncologists, and other doctors to improve outcomes and quality of life.

4. Supportive Care: In addition to cancer-directed therapy, supportive care interventions can assist manage symptoms, alleviate treatment adverse effects, and enhance the quality of life for patients with recurrent bladder cancer. Palliative care services can provide holistic support to meet physical, emotional, and psychosocial needs throughout the cancer experience.

By participating in frequent monitoring, adopting preventative measures, and swiftly addressing any indicators of recurrence, bladder cancer survivors can optimize their health, reduce the chance of cancer recurrence, and enhance overall quality of life.

Chapter 8: Advances in Bladder Cancer Research

Emerging Therapies

Advances in bladder cancer research have led to the development of novel medicines aimed at improving treatment outcomes and quality of life for persons affected by this illness. Emerging therapeutics for bladder cancer comprise different methods, including immunotherapy, targeted therapy, gene therapy, and innovative drug delivery systems. Here are some important developments in bladder cancer research:

1. Immunotherapy: Immunotherapy has emerged as a viable treatment strategy for bladder cancer, particularly for individuals with advanced or metastatic illness. Immune checkpoint inhibitors, such as pembrolizumab, atezolizumab, and nivolumab, target proteins that suppress the immune response, allowing the immune system to recognize and fight cancer cells. These medicines have shown efficacy in improving overall survival and progression-free survival in patients with advanced bladder cancer.

2. Targeted Therapy: Targeted therapy focuses on specific molecular targets implicated in cancer growth and progression. Agents targeting fibroblast growth factor receptor (FGFR) mutations or changes, such as erdafitinib and pemigatinib, have shown promise in clinical trials for treating advanced bladder cancer. Other targeted therapeutics under development include inhibitors of the PI3K/AKT/mTOR pathway and epidermal growth factor receptor (EGFR) inhibitors.

3. Gene Therapy: Gene therapy includes the transfer of genetic material to specific cells to affect their function or behavior. In bladder cancer research, gene therapy approaches aim to limit tumor growth, induce apoptosis (cell death), or improve immune responses to cancer cells. Clinical trials addressing gene therapy for bladder cancer are ongoing, with promising preliminary findings.

4. Novel Drug Delivery Systems: Advancements in drug delivery systems have helped the development of targeted and localized therapy for bladder cancer. Nanoparticle-based drug delivery systems, liposomal formulations, and intravesical drug delivery techniques enable for precision delivery of therapeutic medicines to the bladder while limiting systemic side effects. These novel techniques have the potential to enhance therapeutic efficacy and decrease treatment-related toxicity.

5. Combination medicines: Combination medicines that target several pathways involved in bladder cancer growth and progression are being studied to enhance therapeutic efficacy and overcome resistance mechanisms. Combinations of immunotherapy drugs, targeted treatments, chemotherapy, and radiation therapy are being examined in clinical trials to determine their safety and efficacy in bladder cancer treatment.

Clinical Trials

Clinical trials serve a key role in promoting bladder cancer research by assessing new medicines, developing novel therapeutic techniques, and expanding understanding of the disease biology. Participation in clinical trials allows eligible patients access to cutting-edge medicines and contributes to the progress of scientific knowledge. Here are some major elements of bladder cancer clinical trials:

1. Investigational medicines: Clinical trials may study the safety and efficacy of novel medicines, including immunotherapy drugs, targeted therapies, gene therapy, and combination regimens, for various stages and subtypes of bladder cancer.

2. Patient Eligibility: Eligibility requirements for bladder cancer clinical trials vary depending on factors such as disease stage, previous therapies received, age, performance status, and unique molecular characteristics of the tumor. Your healthcare team can help evaluate if you match the qualifying criteria for a particular clinical trial.

3. Trial Design: Clinical trials may be planned as phase I, phase II, or phase III trials, each serving a different role in testing investigational medicines. Phase I trials analyze safety and determine the optimum dosage of a new medicine, while phase II trials evaluate efficacy and ideal treatment regimes. Phase III trials evaluate the novel therapy to regular treatment or placebo to determine its effectiveness.

4. Informed Consent: Before participating in a clinical study, you will get complete information about the trial, including its goal, potential risks and benefits, treatment procedures, and alternatives. You will be asked to submit informed consent stating your awareness of the trial and desire to participate.

5. Follow-Up and Monitoring: Throughout the research, participants get regular medical monitoring and follow-up evaluations to evaluate therapy response, control adverse effects, and maintain patient safety. Close communication between participants and the research team is vital for the effectiveness of clinical studies.

Developments in bladder cancer research are fast shifting the landscape of bladder cancer treatment and bringing new hope for patients. Emerging medicines, including immunotherapy, targeted therapy, gene therapy, and novel drug delivery systems, hold promise for improving outcomes and quality of life for those affected by this disease. Participation in clinical trials is vital for promoting innovation and accelerating progress in bladder cancer research and therapy.

Chapter 9: Personal Stories of Hope and Resilience

Patient Perspectives

Personal stories of hope and perseverance from bladder cancer patients give inspiration, encouragement, and useful insights into the struggles and successes of living with this disease. Here are some heartwarming narratives from individuals who have confronted bladder cancer with courage and resilience:

1. Jane's Journey: Jane, a lively lady in her 50s, was diagnosed with bladder cancer after having recurrent urine symptoms. Despite the shock of her diagnosis, Jane embraced her treatment with dedication and positivity. She underwent surgery to remove the tumor followed by chemotherapy and immunotherapy. Throughout her journey, Jane found strength in connecting with fellow patients, exchanging experiences, and supporting each other through difficult times. Today, Jane is an outspoken advocate for bladder cancer awareness and empowerment, bringing hope and encouragement to others experiencing similar problems.

2. Mark's Miracle: Mark, a committed husband and father of two, received a tragic diagnosis of advanced bladder cancer at the age of 40. Despite the grave prognosis, Mark refused to give up hope and went on a tough treatment plan that included surgery, chemotherapy, and radiation therapy. Throughout his treatment, Mark took strength from the love and support of his family and friends, as well as his unshakeable faith. Against all chances, Mark's cancer responded to therapy, and he is now cancer-free, cherishing each day as a beautiful gift and sharing his tale of strength with others.

3. Sarah's Survivorship: Sarah, a retired schoolteacher and avid gardener, was diagnosed with non-invasive bladder cancer following a regular check-up. Determined to combat the sickness with grace and tenacity, Sarah underwent many operations and rounds of intravesical therapy to keep the cancer at bay. Despite the physical and emotional toll of her therapy, Sarah remained hopeful and appreciative of each day. She sought refuge in nature, spending time in her garden and finding beauty and inspiration in the simplest of things. Today, Sarah is thriving as a bladder cancer survivor, embracing life with appreciation, resilience, and a fresh sense of purpose.

Caregiver Experiences

Caregivers play a key part in the journey of patients with bladder cancer, delivering love, support, and practical aid during diagnosis, treatment, and recovery. Here are some poignant examples of caregivers who have stuck by their loved ones with steadfast loyalty and compassion:

1. John's Journey as a Caregiver: John, a dedicated husband and caregiver to his wife Mary, was thrown into the job of caregiver after Mary was diagnosed with aggressive bladder cancer. Despite the hardships and uncertainties they faced, John remained by Mary's side every step of the way, offering unfailing support, comfort, and encouragement. He attended doctor's appointments, helped manage prescriptions, and provided emotional support during Mary's most difficult moments. John's devotion and dedication were a source of strength and inspiration to Mary, and together, they navigated the ups and downs of Mary's cancer journey with love and tenacity.

2. Emily's Experience as a Daughter: Emily's mother, Margaret, was diagnosed with bladder cancer while Emily was barely a teenager. As Margaret's principal caregiver, Emily juggled the pressures of school, job, and caring with grace and tenacity. She accompanied her mother to innumerable appointments, offered emotional support during treatment, and helped manage household activities and obligations. Despite the obstacles of caregiving at an early age, Emily stayed persistent in her devotion to her mother's well-being, finding strength in their link and shared love. Margaret's fortitude and tenacity motivated Emily to seek a healthcare career, where she continues to assist and advocate for patients and caregivers experiencing similar struggles.

3. David's Dedication as a Son: David's father, James, confronted bladder cancer with fortitude and determination, accompanied every step of the way by his devoted son. David took on the position of caregiver with humility and compassion, ensuring his father received the best possible care and support throughout his cancer journey. He gave emotional support, helped schedule medical visits, and offered practical aid with daily duties and personal care. Despite the emotional toll of his father's illness, David stayed persistent in his devotion to his father's well-being, cherishing every minute they shared and gaining strength from their bond as father and son.

Personal stories of hope and resilience from bladder cancer patients and caregivers remind us of the ability of the human spirit to overcome adversity, find meaning in tough circumstances, and emerge stronger and more resilient than ever before. These stories serve as beacons of hope and inspiration, bringing encouragement and support to others facing similar problems on their cancer journey.

Conclusion

In conclusion, this book on bladder cancer provides a comprehensive review of the condition, covering numerous areas ranging from comprehending its causes and symptoms to analyzing treatment options, survivorship, and personal stories of hope and resilience. Bladder cancer provides major problems, both for those diagnosed with the disease and their caretakers, but it also reveals the incredible strength and endurance of the human spirit in the face of adversity.

Throughout the pages of this book, readers have obtained insights into the newest breakthroughs in bladder cancer research, including emerging medicines and ongoing clinical trials that show promise for enhancing treatment outcomes and quality of life. By understanding the complexities of bladder cancer and staying informed about advancements in diagnosis, treatment, and supportive care, individuals affected by this disease can empower themselves to make informed decisions, advocate for their health, and navigate their cancer journey with courage and resilience.

Moreover, the personal experiences recounted within these pages serve as a compelling reminder of the human experience behind the statistics and technical nomenclature. From patients who have faced bladder cancer with unflinching tenacity to caregivers who have provided persistent support and love, these narratives inspire hope, create understanding, and underline the significance of compassion and connection in the cancer experience.

As we reflect on the collective wisdom, insights, and experiences presented in this book, let us remember that bladder cancer is not just a diagnosis but a journey—one marked by obstacles, successes, and moments of amazing resilience. By coming together as a community, raising awareness, funding research, and showing compassion to those affected by bladder cancer, we may strive towards a future where every individual diagnosed with this disease can find hope, healing, and a revitalized sense of purpose. Together, we can work towards a world where bladder cancer is not merely treatable but avoidable, and where every survivor's narrative is one of hope, perseverance, and success.

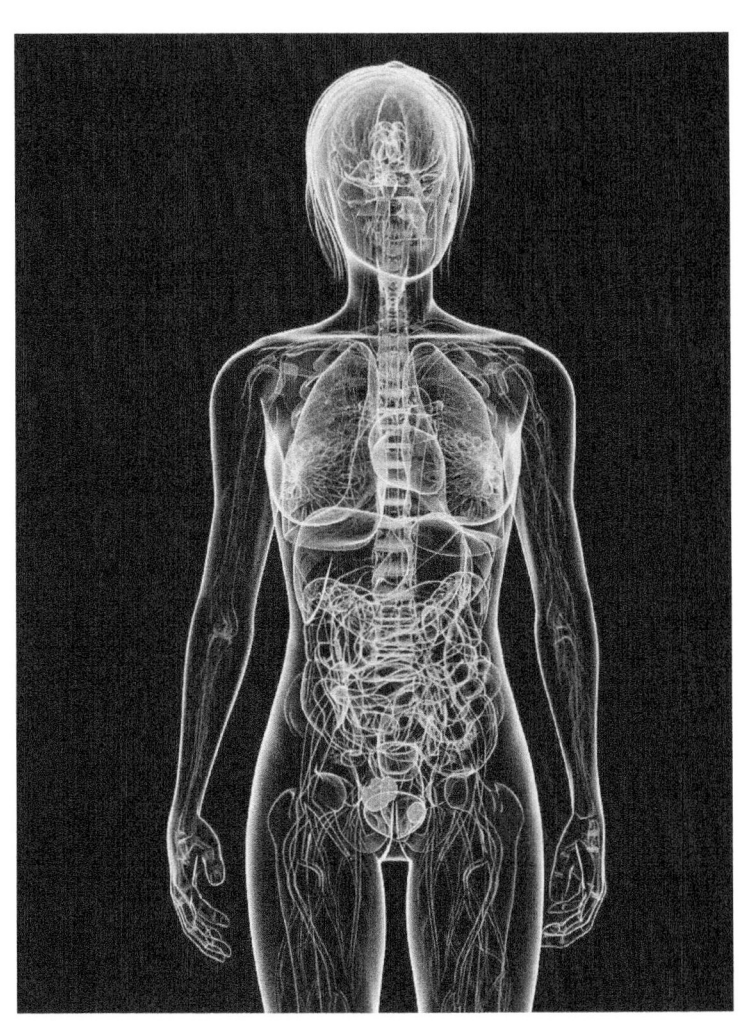

82 | BLADDER CANCER

Printed in Great Britain
by Amazon